The Modern Caveman

Cookbook

A Collection of Paleo Recipes for Busy and
Health-Conscious Individuals

BY

Alex Aton

Licensing Information

It is strictly prohibited to engage in any commercial or non-commercial activity related to the content of this book without the explicit permission of the author. This includes, but is not limited to, selling, publishing, printing, copying, disseminating, or distributing the content in any form or medium. The author holds exclusive rights to the content and reserves the right to take legal action against any unauthorized usage.

If you have obtained an illegal copy of this book, please delete it immediately and obtain a legal version. Purchasing a legal version of this book supports the author's hard work and dedication in creating the content.

However, the author does not take responsibility for any actions taken by the reader based on the information provided in the book. The content is intended solely as an informational tool and the author has taken all necessary steps to ensure its accuracy. However, as with any information source, caution must be exercised when taking any steps based on the content of this book. It is advisable to seek professional guidance before taking any significant actions based on the information provided in this book.

Table of Contents

Introduction

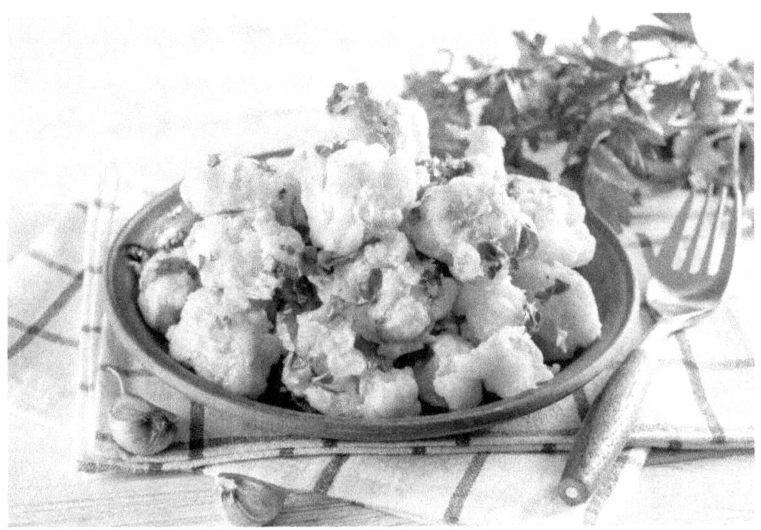

Welcome to a culinary adventure that takes you back in time while embracing the best of the modern world - "The Modern Caveman Cookbook." Within these pages, you will find a collection of delicious and nutritious recipes that celebrate the Paleo diet, a way of eating that is known for its health benefits and emphasis on whole, real foods.

So, whether you're a seasoned Paleo believer or new to the lifestyle, "The Modern Caveman Cookbook" has something for you. Get ready to discover a new world of flavors and textures, and take the first step towards a healthier, happier you.

XXXXXXXXXXXXXXXXXXXXX

1. Baked Avocado Eggs

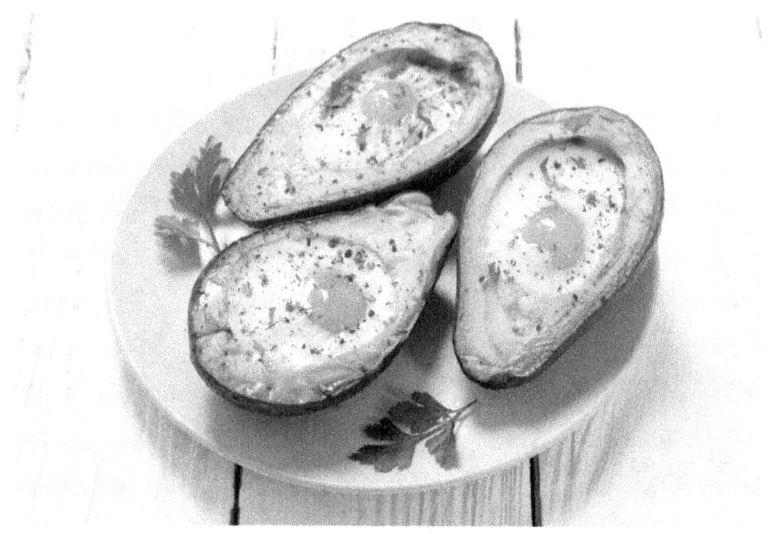

Creamy, buttery, and packed with protein, our baked avocado eggs are a delicious and healthy meal option. Made by baking ripe avocados filled with eggs, this recipe is flavorful and easy to make. Satisfy your cravings with a breakfast that is low in carbs and high in nutrients.

Preparation Time: 25 min.

Serving Size: 2

Ingredients:

- 2 avocados
- 4 eggs
- Salt
- Pepper

xxxxxxxxxxxxxxxxxxxxxx

Instructions:

a) Start by preheating your oven to 425°F (220°C).

b) Cut the avocados in half and carefully remove the pits.

c) To create a slightly larger cavity, scoop out a small amount of flesh from each avocado half.

d) Arrange the prepared avocado halves in a baking dish.

e) Carefully crack one egg into each avocado half.

f) Season with salt and pepper to your taste preference.

g) Bake your avocado and egg creations in the preheated oven for approximately 15-20 minutes, or until the eggs reach your desired level of doneness.

h) Once done, remove from the oven and allow them to cool for a few minutes before serving.

Cooking Notes:

- You can get creative with toppings by adding ingredients like shredded cheese, chopped herbs, or crumbled bacon before baking for added flavor and texture.
- For a spicy kick, consider adding a pinch of cayenne pepper or a dash of hot sauce on top of the eggs before baking.
- To ensure the eggs cook evenly, you can make a small indentation in the avocado flesh before cracking the egg into it; this will help prevent the egg from spilling over the sides.
- If you prefer a runny yolk, aim for the shorter end of the baking time, around 15 minutes, while those who prefer a firmer yolk can go closer to 20 minutes.
- Ensure the avocados are stable in the baking dish to prevent any tipping over during cooking.
- These Baked Avocado Eggs are a versatile dish and can be enjoyed as a simple breakfast or a satisfying brunch option.

2. Paleo Chia Seed Pudding

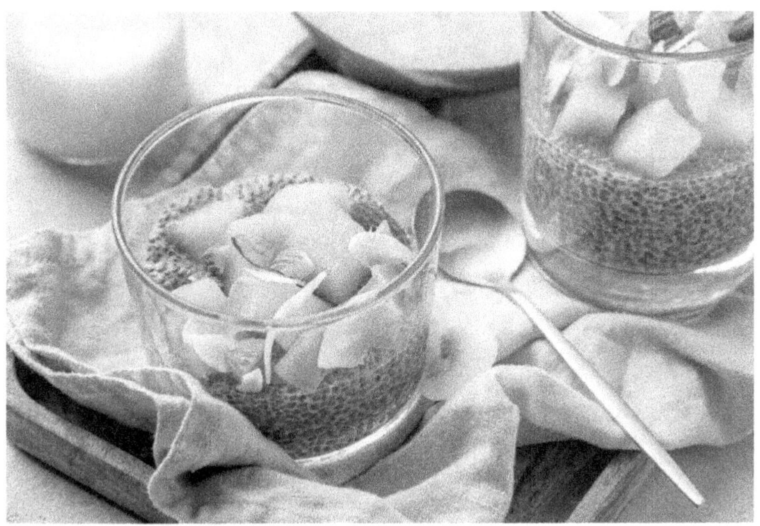

Indulge in a sweet and satisfying treat with our Paleo Chia Seed Pudding. Made with natural ingredients like coconut milk, chia seeds, and honey, this recipe is a healthy and delicious dessert or snack option. Enjoy it guilt-free as a low-sugar, nutrient-dense alternative to traditional pudding.

Preparation Time: 25 min.

Serving Size: 2

Ingredients:

- 1/4 cup of chia seeds
- 1 cup of coconut milk
- 1 tablespoon of honey
- 1/2 teaspoon of vanilla extract

XXXXXXXXXXXXXXXXXXXXXX

Instructions:

a) In a bowl, combine chia seeds, coconut milk, honey, and vanilla extract, whisking them together thoroughly.

b) Allow the mixture to rest for 5 minutes, then whisk again to ensure there are no clumps of chia seeds.

c) Cover the bowl and refrigerate it for a minimum of 20 minutes, or until the pudding reaches the desired thickness.

d) Serve your Chia Seed Pudding in individual bowls or glasses, and embellish with your preferred toppings, such as fresh berries or nuts.

Cooking Notes:

- Chia seed pudding can be refrigerated for several hours or overnight for a thicker consistency and enhanced flavor.

- To add a delightful crunch and extra nutrients to your pudding, consider topping it with a sprinkle of toasted coconut flakes, chopped almonds, or pecans.

- If you prefer a smoother pudding texture, you can blend the mixture in a blender or food processor before refrigerating it. This will break down the chia seeds and create a creamier consistency.

- For a fun twist, layer the chia seed pudding with alternating layers of fruit compote or jam to create a parfait-style dessert.

- Feel free to experiment with different sweeteners or flavorings, like maple syrup or cocoa powder, to personalize your pudding.

- Chia seeds absorb liquid, so don't be alarmed if the pudding appears runny at first; it will thicken as it sits in the refrigerator.

3. Low-Calorie Protein Smoothies

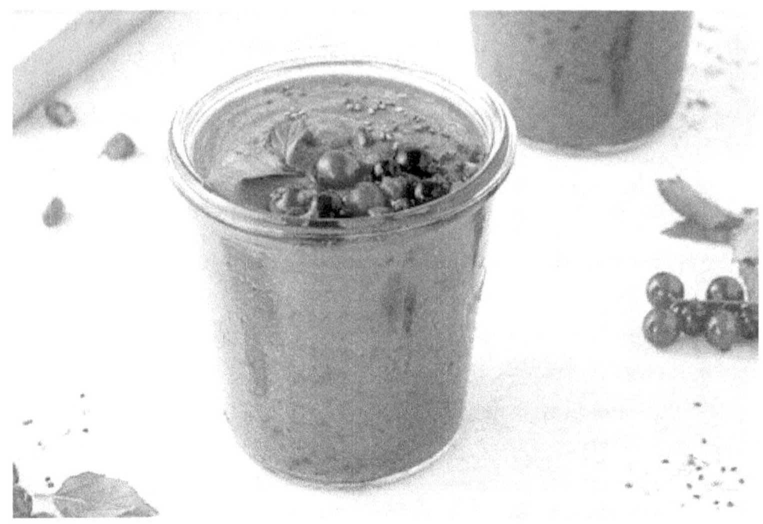

Stay healthy and energized with our Low-Calorie Protein Smoothies. Packed with nutritious superfoods like fruits, veggies, and protein, these smoothies are a perfect meal replacement or snack option. Satisfy your cravings while keeping calories in check with our delicious and refreshing smoothie recipes.

Preparation Time: 15 min.

Serving Size: 2

Ingredients:

- 2 cups of unsweetened almond milk
- 1 scoop of protein powder
- 1 cup of frozen berries
- 1 tablespoon of almond butter
- 1 tablespoon of chia seeds

XXXXXXXXXXXXXXXXXXXXXX

Instructions:

a) Begin by placing all the ingredients into a blender.

b) Blend the mixture until it becomes smooth and reaches a creamy consistency.

c) Pour the smoothie into serving glasses and savor its deliciousness.

Cooking Notes:

- Customize your low-calorie protein smoothie by experimenting with different types of protein powder flavors or adding spinach or kale for an extra boost of nutrients.
- Adjust the thickness of your smoothie by adding more or less almond milk to suit your preference.
- To make your low-calorie protein smoothie even more filling, you can add a handful of rolled oats or a spoonful of Greek yogurt for added fiber and creaminess.
- Don't forget that you can incorporate vegetables like spinach, kale, or cucumber into your smoothies without significantly affecting the calorie count while boosting their nutritional value.
- If you're using fresh fruits instead of frozen ones, you can add a few ice cubes to your blender to make the smoothie colder and more refreshing.
- For a sweeter taste, you can include a drizzle of honey or maple syrup.

4. Baked Ham and Egg Cups

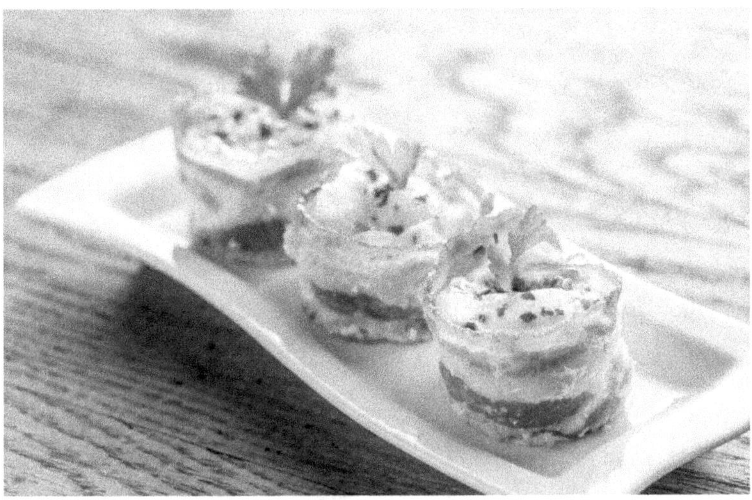

Enjoy a classic breakfast dish with a twist - our Baked Ham and Egg Cups. Made with savory ham and filled with protein-packed eggs, this recipe is a flavorful and easy-to-make meal option. Perfect for busy mornings, these cups are a delicious and satisfying breakfast that will keep you energized throughout the day.

Preparation Time: 35 min.

Serving Size: 4

Ingredients:

- 4 slices of ham
- 4 eggs

XXXXXXXXXXXXXXXXXXXXXX

Instructions:

a) Begin by preheating your oven to 375°F (190°C).

b) Grease a muffin tin generously with cooking spray to prevent sticking.

c) Line each muffin cup with a slice of ham, creating a ham "cup" to hold the egg.

d) Carefully crack one egg into each of the ham-lined cups.

e) Place the muffin tin in the preheated oven and bake for approximately 15-20 minutes or until the eggs reach your preferred level of doneness.

f) Once done, take the baked ham and egg cups out of the oven, and allow them to cool for a few minutes before serving.

Cooking Notes:

- You can personalize these baked ham and egg cups by adding ingredients like shredded cheese, diced vegetables, or herbs before cracking the eggs for extra flavor and texture.

- Ensure that the ham slices overlap the edges of each muffin cup to create a sturdy "cup" to hold the egg.

- For added flavor and variety, consider incorporating ingredients like shredded cheddar or Swiss cheese, diced bell peppers, diced tomatoes, chopped spinach, or even cooked bacon bits into the ham cups before adding the eggs. These additions can complement the savory ham and provide a burst of flavor in each bite.

- To ensure the ham slices fit neatly into the muffin cups and create a secure "cup" shape, you can trim the edges of the ham slices with kitchen scissors or a knife, if necessary. This will help create a uniform and visually appealing final dish.

- These cups make a convenient and protein-packed breakfast or brunch option, and they can be easily prepared in advance and reheated when needed.

5. Baked Eggs with Parma Ham in Portobello Mushroom Cups

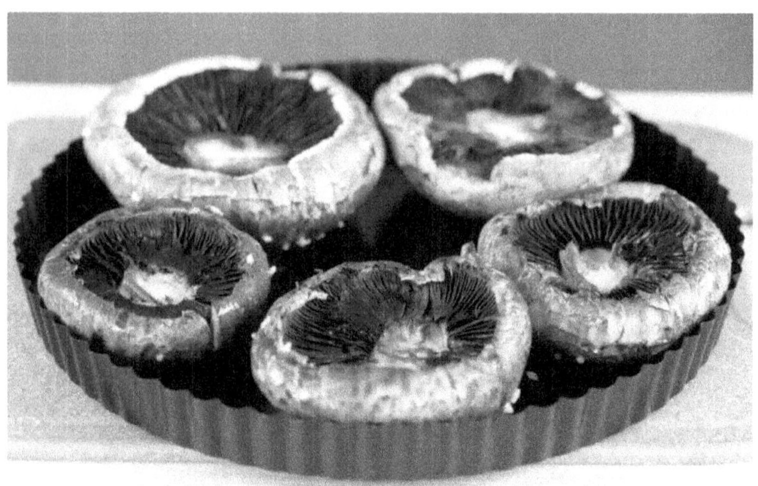

Elevate breakfast with Baked Eggs & Parma Ham in Portobello Mushroom Cups. Packed with protein, the savory ham & mushroom combo promises a tasty and healthy morning meal.

Preparation Time: 35 min.

Serving Size: 4

Ingredients:

- 4 Portobello mushrooms
- 4 slices of Parma ham
- 4 eggs
- Pepper and Salt to taste

xxxxxxxxxxxxxxxxxxxx

Instructions:

a) Start by preheating your oven to 375°F.

b) Begin preparing the Portobello mushrooms by removing their stems and gently scraping off the gills using a spoon.

c) Place the cleaned mushroom caps on a baking sheet lined with parchment paper.

d) Season the mushroom caps with salt and pepper for added flavor.

e) Wrap each mushroom cap with a delicate, thin slice of Parma ham, ensuring it encases the mushroom entirely.

f) Carefully crack one egg into the center of each mushroom cap.

g) Bake your assembled mushroom cups in the preheated oven for approximately 20-25 minutes or until the eggs reach your desired level of doneness.

h) Once done, take the baked eggs with Parma ham in Portobello mushroom cups out of the oven and allow them to cool for a few minutes before serving.

Cooking Notes:

- To prevent the mushrooms from releasing excess moisture during baking, you can lightly brush them with olive oil before seasoning.

- When selecting Portobello mushrooms for this dish, choose ones that are firm and without any signs of moisture or mold. Fresh mushrooms with a smooth cap work best for holding the egg and ham.

- To ensure that the eggs are cooked to your liking, you can check their doneness by gently tapping the egg yolks with a fork or knife. For runny yolks, aim for about 10-12 minutes of baking, while longer baking times, up to 15 minutes or more, will result in firmer yolks.

- Experiment with different herbs or grated cheese for added flavor variations.

- These baked eggs are a delightful and protein-packed breakfast or brunch option, and they pair beautifully with a side salad or toasted bread.

6. Sausage and Egg Sandwich

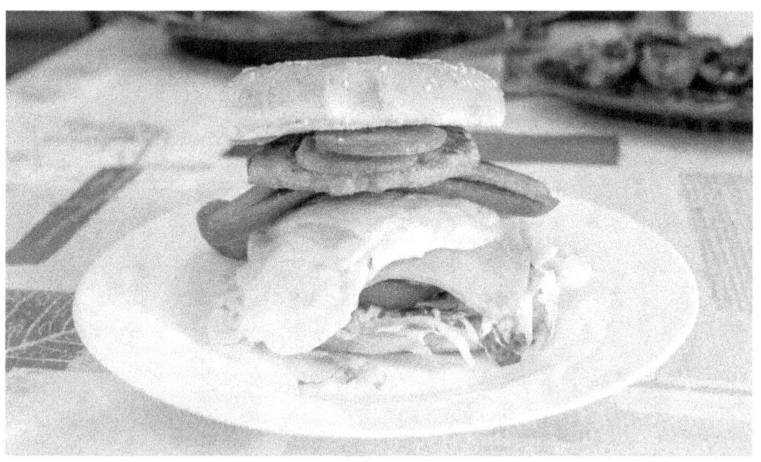

Start your day off right with our savory Sausage and Egg Sandwich. Made with a freshly toasted English muffin, a juicy sausage patty and topped with a perfectly cooked egg, this breakfast sandwich packs a protein punch to keep you fueled all morning long. Satisfy your breakfast cravings and enjoy this delicious breakfast option on the go.

Preparation Time: 35 min.

Serving Size: 4

Ingredients:

- 4 sausages
- 4 eggs
- 8 slices of bread
- 4 slices of cheese
- Butter or oil for cooking

xxxxxxxxxxxxxxxxxxxxxx

Instructions:

a) Begin by preheating a frying pan over medium heat.

b) Cook the sausages in the frying pan until they turn browned and are cooked through, which usually takes about 10 minutes.

c) While the sausages are cooking, crack the eggs into a bowl and lightly beat them with a fork.

d) Heat another frying pan or use the same one after removing the sausages. Add butter or oil to the pan.

e) Pour the beaten eggs into the pan and cook them until they are fully set, stirring occasionally to achieve a fluffy texture.

f) Toast the slices of bread in a toaster or on a separate pan.

g) Assemble each sandwich by placing a cooked sausage, a slice of cheese, and a portion of scrambled egg between two slices of toast.

h) Repeat this process for the remaining sandwiches.

i) Serve your freshly made sausage and egg sandwiches while they are hot and savor the deliciousness.

Cooking Notes:

- Customize your sandwich by adding condiments like ketchup, hot sauce, or mayonnaise for extra flavor.
- For a healthier option, consider using turkey or chicken sausages instead of pork sausages. They are lower in fat and calories while still providing great flavor.
- To make your scrambled eggs even creamier, you can add a splash of milk or cream to the beaten eggs before cooking.
- You can also include additional toppings such as lettuce, tomato slices, or avocado for added freshness and texture.
- These sandwiches make for a quick and hearty breakfast, brunch, or even a satisfying meal on the go.

7. Coconut Flour Pancakes

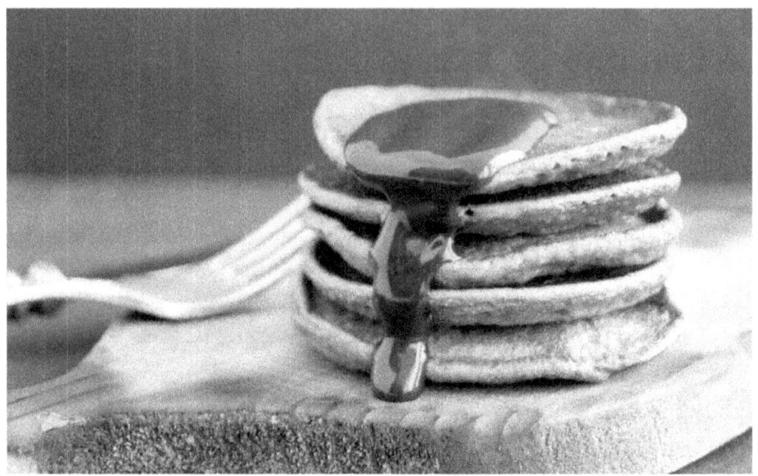

Experience a gluten-free delight with our Coconut Flour Pancakes. Made with wholesome ingredients, these fluffy and flavorful pancakes are a breakfast favorite. Enjoy a stack drizzled in maple syrup for a delicious and guilt-free morning treat.

Preparation Time: 25 min.

Serving Size: 2

Ingredients:

- 1/4 cup of coconut flour
- 4 eggs
- 1/4 cup of almond milk
- 1 tsp of baking powder
- 1 tsp of vanilla extract
- 1 tbsp of honey
- 1/4 cup of shredded coconut
- Coconut oil for cooking

XXXXXXXXXXXXXXXXXXXXXX

Instructions:

a) Start by whisking together in a mixing bowl: coconut flour, eggs, almond milk, baking powder, vanilla extract, and honey until they are thoroughly combined.

b) Add the shredded coconut to the mixture and stir it in.

c) Heat a non-stick pan over medium heat and lightly brush it with coconut oil.

d) Pour 1/4 cup of pancake batter onto the pan for each pancake.

e) Cook each pancake for 2-3 minutes on each side, or until they turn a delightful golden brown.

f) Serve the warm pancakes with your choice of toppings, such as fresh fruit, maple syrup, or yogurt.

Cooking Notes:

- Coconut flour tends to absorb more liquid than regular flour, so the batter may be thicker. If it's too thick, you can add a bit more almond milk to achieve your desired consistency.
- Be patient when flipping the pancakes; they can be delicate, so use a spatula gently.
- Customize your pancakes by adding chocolate chips, blueberries, or nuts to the batter for extra flavor and texture.
- When working with coconut flour, allow the batter to sit for a few minutes before cooking. This gives the flour time to absorb the liquid and helps achieve a better texture.
- To keep the pancakes warm while cooking batches, you can place them on a baking sheet in a low oven (around 200°F or 93°C) until you're ready to serve.
- Adjust the sweetness by varying the amount of honey or using alternative sweeteners like maple syrup or agave nectar.

8. Baked Avocado Fries

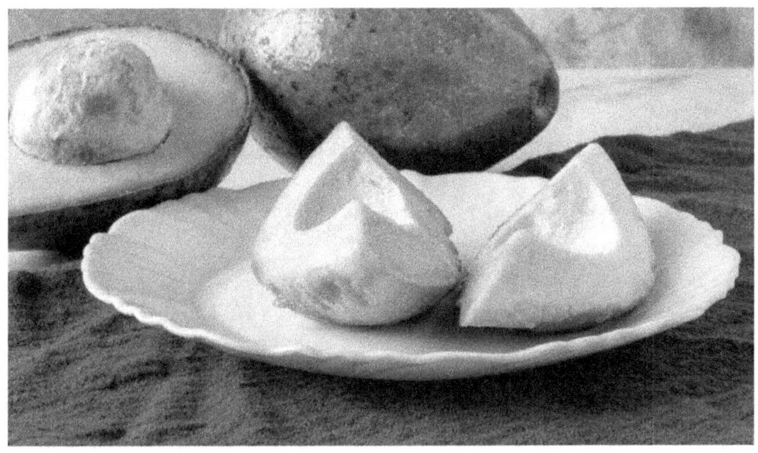

Indulge in a healthy snack with our Baked Avocado Fries. Creamy avocado slices are coated in a golden and crispy crust, delivering a satisfying crunch in each bite. Enjoy guilt-free snacking with this nutritious twist on classic French fries.

Preparation Time: 25 min.

Serving Size: 2

Ingredients:

- 2 avocados
- 1 cup of bread crumbs
- 1/2 teaspoon of paprika
- 1/2 teaspoon of garlic powder
- 1/4 teaspoon of salt
- 1/4 teaspoon of black pepper
- 2 eggs, beaten

xxxxxxxxxxxxxxxxxxxxxx

Instructions:

a) Begin by preheating your oven to 425°F (220°C) and lining a baking sheet with parchment paper.

b) Take the avocados, cut them in half, remove the pit, and slice each half into 4-5 wedges.

c) In a bowl, combine the bread crumbs, paprika, salt, garlic powder, and black pepper.

d) Dip each avocado slice into a beaten egg, ensuring it's well-coated, and then coat it with the breadcrumb mixture.

e) Arrange the coated avocado slices on the prepared baking sheet.

f) Bake in the preheated oven for 15-20 minutes, or until the fries achieve a delightful golden brown and crispy texture.

g) Serve these scrumptious baked avocado fries while they're hot, alongside your preferred dipping sauce.

Cooking Notes:

- Use ripe but firm avocados for the best results.
- To make the fries extra crispy, you can lightly spray or drizzle them with oil before baking.
- Experiment with different dipping sauces like ranch dressing, salsa, or chipotle mayo to enhance the flavor.
- If you prefer a spicier kick, consider adding a pinch of cayenne pepper or chili powder to the breadcrumb mixture.
- For an even lighter version of these avocado fries, you can use whole-grain bread crumbs or panko breadcrumbs.
- These avocado fries are best when served immediately, as they tend to lose their crispiness over time.
- These fries are a healthier alternative to traditional potato fries, offering a creamy interior and a satisfying crunch. Enjoy!

9. Gluten-Free Egg Muffins

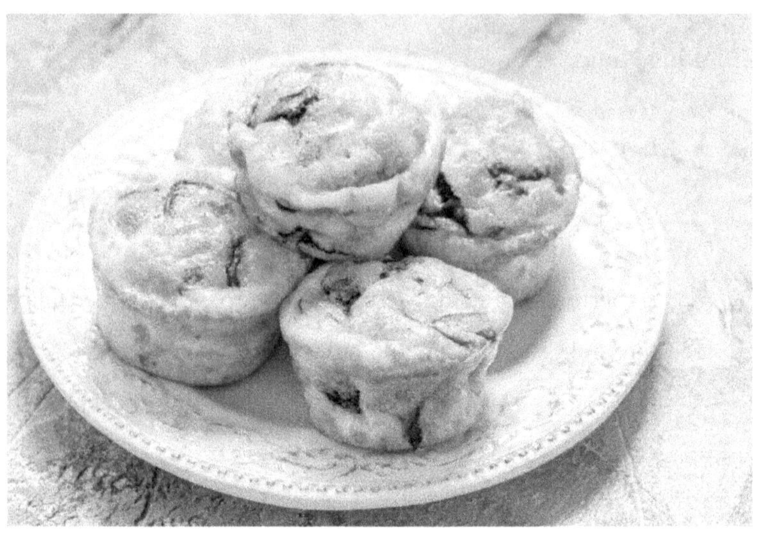

Start your morning with our Gluten-Free Egg Muffins. Packed with protein and veggies, these perfectly portioned muffins are a convenient and healthy breakfast option. Enjoy them hot or cold for a delicious and satisfying meal on the go.

Preparation Time: 15 min.

Serving Size: 2

Ingredients:

- 6 eggs
- 1/4 cup of milk
- 1/4 cup of diced vegetables (e.g.bell peppers, onions, spinach)
- Salt and pepper

xxxxxxxxxxxxxxxxxxxxxx

Instructions:

a) Begin by preheating your oven to 350°F.

b) In a mixing bowl, beat together the eggs and milk until well combined.

c) Add the diced vegetables, salt, and pepper to the egg mixture, and stir thoroughly.

d) Grease the muffin pans with cooking spray or oil to prevent sticking.

e) Evenly pour the egg mixture into the muffin tin cups.

f) Bake in the preheated oven for 12-15 minutes or until the muffins are set and have a slight golden hue on top.

g) After removing them from the oven, allow the egg muffins to cool for 1-2 minutes.

h) Carefully take out the egg muffins from the muffin tin.

i) Serve these delectable gluten-free egg muffins while they are warm and savor the flavors.

Cooking Notes:

- Feel free to experiment with your choice of vegetables, cheese, or herbs to create a variety of flavors in your egg muffins.

- If you'd like to add cheese to your egg muffins, sprinkle some grated cheese on top of each muffin cup before baking. Cheddar, feta, or mozzarella work well with this recipe.

- To check if the egg muffins are fully cooked, insert a toothpick into the center of one; if it comes out clean, they're done.

- You can also add cooked bacon bits, sausage, or diced ham for a meatier version of these egg muffins.

- These muffins are excellent for meal prep. Store them in an airtight container in the refrigerator for a convenient grab-and-go breakfast or snack option.

- Ensure not to overfill the muffin cups to prevent overflow during baking.

10. Paleo Egg Drop Soup

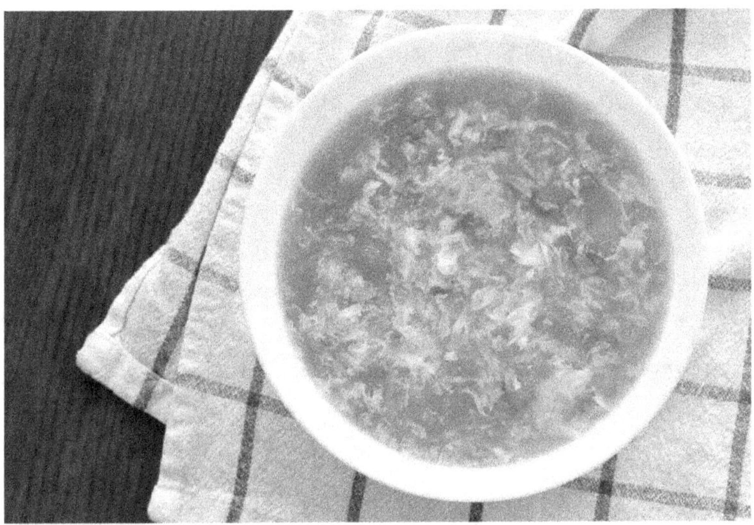

Experience a comforting bowl of Paleo Egg Drop Soup. Made with nourishing bone broth, this warm and savory soup is filled with delicate egg ribbons and flavorful herbs. Enjoy this gluten-free and dairy-free option for a light yet satisfying meal.

Preparation Time: 25 min.

Serving Size: 2

Ingredients:

- 4 cups of chicken broth
- 4 eggs
- 2 green onions
- 1/2 teaspoon of salt
- 1/4 teaspoon of ground black pepper

xxxxxxxxxxxxxxxxxxxxxx

Instructions:

a) Start by bringing the chicken broth to a boil in a pot.

b) In a separate bowl, whisk the eggs.

c) As the broth simmers, stir it in circular motions and slowly pour in the beaten egg to create delicate ribbons.

d) Next, introduce the chopped green onions, salt, and black pepper to the soup.

e) Let the soup simmer for 5 minutes to allow the flavors to meld together.

f) Serve the Paleo Egg Drop Soup piping hot.

Cooking Notes:

- You can add other ingredients like sliced mushrooms, spinach, or cooked chicken for extra texture and flavor.
- Be cautious when adding salt, as the chicken broth may already contain sodium. Adjust to your taste preference.
- To enhance the flavor, consider adding a dash of coconut aminos or fish sauce for an umami boost, which complements the richness of the bone broth.
- If you prefer a thicker consistency, you can mix a teaspoon of arrowroot flour or tapioca starch with a bit of cold water and then add it to the soup, stirring well until it thickens.
- This soup is an excellent option for a quick and comforting meal, especially on chilly days. Enjoy!

11. Pumpkin Cream Soup

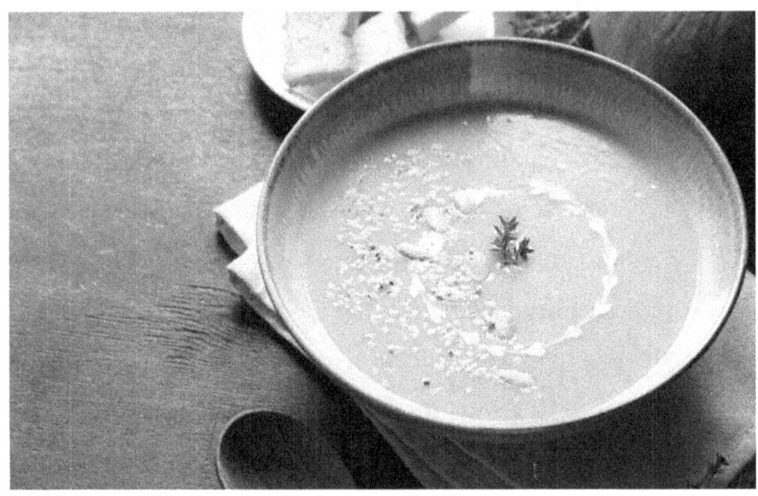

Cozy up with a bowl of our Pumpkin Cream Soup. Made with rich and creamy coconut milk and savory spices, this seasonal soup is bursting with flavor and warmth. Enjoy a comforting and nourishing meal with this gluten-free and vegan option.

Preparation Time: 25 min.

Serving Size: 2

Ingredients:

- 1 small pumpkin
- 1 onion
- 2 cloves of garlic
- 2 cups of vegetable broth
- 1 cup of heavy cream
- Salt and pepper to taste

XXXXXXXXXXXXXXXXXXXXX

Instructions:

a) Begin by cutting the pumpkin in half and removing the seeds.

b) Proceed to peel and chop the onion and garlic cloves.

c) In a pot, sauté the onion and garlic until they turn a golden brown hue.

d) Add the pumpkin to the pot and cook for a few minutes.

e) Pour in the vegetable broth and bring it to a boil. Reduce the heat and let it simmer for about 15 minutes, or until the pumpkin becomes tender.

f) Use a blender to puree the soup until it achieves a smooth consistency. Exercise caution as the soup will be hot.

g) Return the smooth soup to the pot and stir in the heavy cream. Season it with salt and pepper according to your taste.

h) Continue to cook for an additional 5 minutes, occasionally stirring.

i) Serve the Pumpkin Cream Soup while it's hot, and savor the delicious flavors.

Cooking Notes:

- To enhance the flavor, consider adding a pinch of nutmeg or a sprinkle of cinnamon to the soup while cooking.
- For added richness, you can substitute coconut milk for the heavy cream to maintain the vegan and dairy-free qualities of the soup.
- If you find it challenging to cut and peel the pumpkin, you can also roast it in the oven until it's soft and easily scoopable. This can save time and effort while intensifying the pumpkin's flavor.
- Garnish your pumpkin soup with a dollop of sour cream, croutons, or a sprinkle of fresh herbs like parsley or chives for extra texture and presentation.
- This creamy pumpkin soup makes a delightful appetizer or a comforting meal on a chilly day. Enjoy!

12. Paleo Chicken Soup

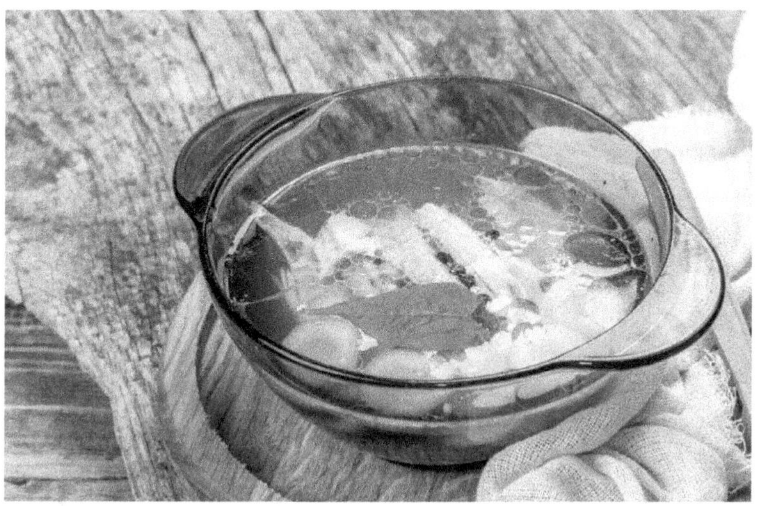

Nourish your body with our Paleo Chicken Soup. Tender chicken simmered in a flavorful broth with vibrant vegetables, this comforting soup is packed with protein and nutrients. Savor the goodness of this gluten-free and dairy-free option for a satisfying meal.

Preparation Time: 25 min.

Serving Size: 2

Ingredients:

- 2 chicken breasts
- 4 cups of chicken broth
- 1 onion
- 2 carrots
- 2 celery stalks
- 2 cloves of garlic
- 1 tsp of dried thyme
- 1 tsp of dried oregano
- Salt and pepper to taste

XXXXXXXXXXXXXXXXXXXXXX

Instructions:

a) Begin by bringing the chicken broth to a boil in a pot.

b) Add chicken breasts, onion, carrots, celery, thyme, garlic, oregano, salt, and pepper to the pot.

c) Reduce the heat to medium and allow the soup to simmer for approximately 20 minutes, or until the chicken is thoroughly cooked.

d) After cooking, remove the chicken breast from the pot and use two forks to shred it into bite-sized pieces.

e) Return the shredded chicken to the pot and stir it into the soup to distribute the flavors evenly.

f) Serve this hearty Paleo Chicken Soup while it's hot and relish the comforting taste.

Cooking Notes:

- For added depth of flavor, consider using bone-in, skin-on chicken breasts or thighs. Remove the skin before shredding the meat.
- To add even more flavor to your Paleo Chicken Soup, you can start by browning the chicken breasts in a hot skillet before adding them to the boiling broth. This step enhances the richness of the soup.
- If you prefer a thicker consistency, you can add a small amount of arrowroot powder or tapioca starch mixed with cold water to the soup. This will act as a natural thickener.
- Feel free to add extra vegetables like spinach, zucchini, or cauliflower for added nutrition and variety.
- This homemade chicken soup is not only delicious but also a soothing option when you're feeling under the weather or in need of warmth and comfort. Enjoy!

13. Creamy Carrot Soup

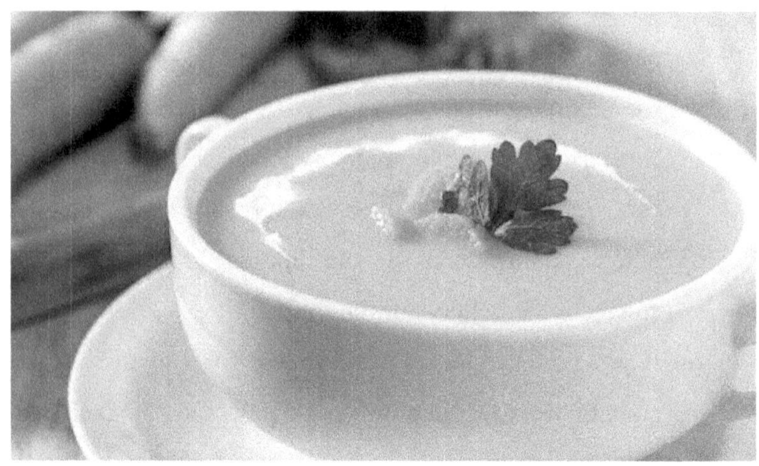

Indulge in the velvety goodness of our Creamy Carrot Soup. Made with fresh carrots and a touch of cream, this wholesome soup is delightfully smooth and bursting with flavor. Treat yourself to this gluten-free and vegetarian option for a comforting and satisfying meal.

Preparation Time: 25 min.

Serving Size: 2

Ingredients:

- 500g carrots
- 1 onion
- 2 cloves of garlic
- 1 tbsp of olive oil
- 500ml of vegetable broth
- 150ml of coconut milk
- Salt and pepper to taste

XXXXXXXXXXXXXXXXXXXXXX

Instructions:

a) Start by peeling and chopping the carrots, onion, and garlic.

b) Heat olive oil in a pot over medium heat.

c) Add the chopped carrots, onion, and garlic to the pot, and sauté them for 5 minutes.

d) Pour in the vegetable broth and bring it to a boil.

e) Reduce the heat to low and let the mixture simmer for approximately 15 minutes, or until the carrots become tender.

f) Remove the pot from the heat and allow it to cool slightly.

g) Use a blender to puree the soup until it achieves a creamy and smooth consistency.

h) Return the pureed soup to the pot and stir in the coconut milk.

i) Season the soup with salt and pepper to taste.

j) Reheat the soup over low heat until it is warmed through.

k) Serve this velvety Creamy Carrot Soup while it's hot and relish its delightful flavors.

Cooking Notes:

- If you prefer a thinner consistency, you can add more vegetable broth or coconut milk.

- To add an extra layer of flavor, you can roast the carrots in the oven before adding them to the soup. Simply toss the chopped carrots with a bit of olive oil and roast them at 400°F (200°C) for about 20-25 minutes or until they are caramelized and tender. This roasting process enhances the natural sweetness of the carrots.

- If you want to make this soup completely vegan, you can substitute the coconut milk with almond milk or another non-dairy milk of your choice. This will give it a slightly different flavor profile but still maintain a creamy consistency.

- Garnish your soup with a sprinkle of fresh herbs like parsley or a swirl of coconut cream for extra flavor and presentation.

- This soup makes for a comforting and nutritious meal, perfect for any season. Enjoy!

14. Grilled Shrimp with Pesto Sauce

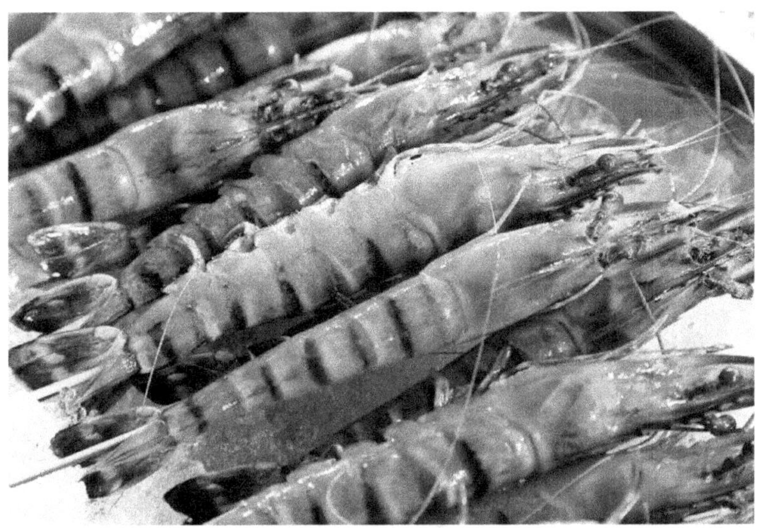

Savor the exquisite flavors of our Grilled Shrimp with Pesto Sauce. Succulent grilled shrimp perfectly paired with a vibrant pesto sauce, this dish is a delightful combination of freshness and tanginess. Enjoy this gluten-free and dairy-free option for a tasty and satisfying meal.

Preparation Time: 25 min.

Serving Size: 4

Ingredients:

- 1 lb. of shrimp, peeled and deveined
- 1/4 cup of pesto sauce
- Salt and pepper to taste

xxxxxxxxxxxxxxxxxxxxxxx

Instructions:

a) Begin by preheating your grill to medium-high heat.

b) Season the shrimp with salt and pepper.

c) Thread the seasoned shrimp on skewers for grilling.

d) Grill the shrimp for approximately 2-3 minutes per side, ensuring they are thoroughly cooked.

e) During the final minute of grilling, brush the shrimp with pesto sauce to infuse flavor.

f) After grilling, carefully remove the shrimp from the grill.

g) Serve your Grilled Shrimp with Pesto Sauce while they are hot and ready to be enjoyed.

Cooking Notes:

- Soak wooden skewers in water for about 30 minutes before using them to prevent them from burning on the grill.

- Grilled shrimp cook quickly, so keep a close eye on them to prevent overcooking. Shrimp are done when they turn pink and opaque. Overcooked shrimp can become rubbery and less flavorful.

- When using wooden skewers, make sure to soak them in water for about 30 minutes before threading the shrimp. This prevents the skewers from catching fire or burning on the grill.

- If using frozen shrimp, thaw them before grilling and pat them dry with paper towels for better grilling results.

- You can prepare your homemade pesto sauce or use store-bought pesto for convenience.

- Grilled shrimp with pesto sauce makes for a delicious appetizer or a delightful addition to a summer meal. Enjoy!

15. Fried Cauliflower

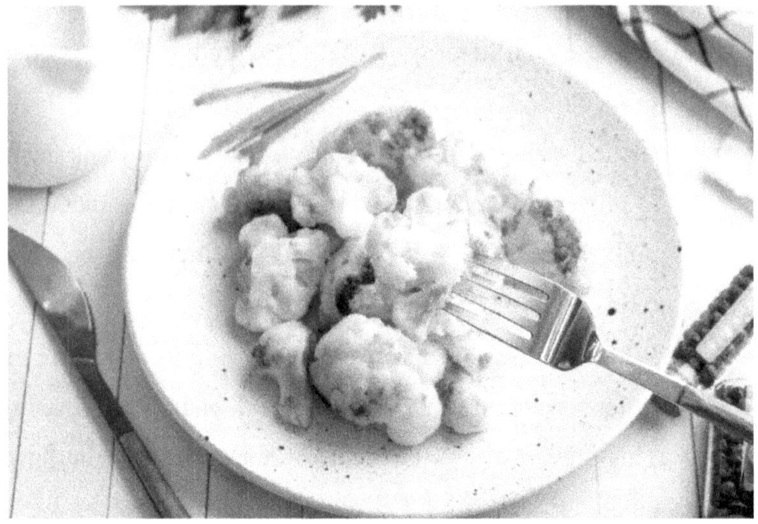

Discover the crispy perfection of our Fried Cauliflower. Lightly battered and fried to a golden brown, this dish offers a delightful crunch with a tender interior. Indulge in this gluten-free and vegan option for a flavorful and guilt-free indulgence.

Preparation Time: 15 min.

Serving Size: 2

Ingredients:

- 1 medium-sized cauliflower
- 2 tablespoons of vegetable oil
- Salt to taste
- Pepper to taste

xxxxxxxxxxxxxxxxxxxxxxx

Instructions:

a) Start by cutting the cauliflower into small florets.

b) Heat vegetable oil in a frying pan over medium heat.

c) Add the cauliflower florets to the pan and season them with salt and pepper.

d) Cook for approximately 10-12 minutes, making sure to stir occasionally, until the cauliflower turns golden brown and achieves a crispy texture.

e) Once done, remove the cauliflower from the heat.

f) Serve your Fried Cauliflower while it's hot and ready to enjoy.

Cooking Notes:

- Be cautious when adding the cauliflower to the hot oil to avoid splatters.
- You can customize the seasoning by adding spices like paprika, garlic powder, or cayenne pepper for extra flavor.
- To test if the oil is hot enough for frying, you can drop a small piece of cauliflower into the oil. If it sizzles and starts to turn golden brown, the oil is ready.
- When frying cauliflower, it's important not to overcrowd the pan. Frying in batches allows the cauliflower to cook evenly and become crispy.
- For a healthier alternative, you can bake the cauliflower in the oven instead of frying it.
- Fried cauliflower makes for a tasty side dish or snack. Enjoy!

16. Egg Cream Salad

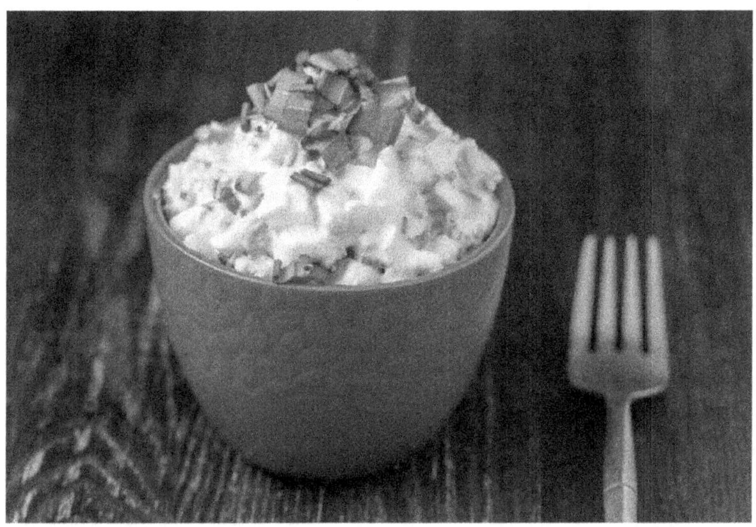

Indulge in the delightful simplicity of our Egg Cream Salad. Creamy eggs paired with a light dressing, this salad offers a blend of textures and flavors. Enjoy this vegetarian and gluten-free option for a refreshing and satisfying dish.

Preparation Time: 25 min.

Serving Size: 2

Ingredients:

- 2 boiled eggs
- 1/4 cup of mayonnaise
- 1/4 cup of sour cream
- 1/4 cup of chopped green onions
- 1/4 cup of chopped celery
- 1/4 teaspoon of Dijon mustard
- Salt and pepper to taste

XXXXXXXXXXXXXXXXXXXXXX

Instructions:

a) Start by mashing the boiled eggs in a bowl using a fork.

b) Add mayonnaise, sour cream, green onions, celery, Dijon mustard, salt, and pepper to the mashed eggs. Ensure thorough mixing.

c) Refrigerate the salad until it's chilled and ready to serve.

Cooking Notes:

- Customize your egg cream salad by adding ingredients like diced pickles, capers, or fresh herbs for extra flavor and texture.
- For added freshness and a burst of color, consider garnishing your Egg Cream Salad with some chopped fresh parsley or chives just before serving.
- You can make this salad ahead of time and refrigerate it for a few hours or even overnight to allow the flavors to meld and develop further.
- This salad is versatile and can be served as a side dish, on sandwiches, or as a topping for crackers. Enjoy its creamy and savory goodness!

17. Taco Pie

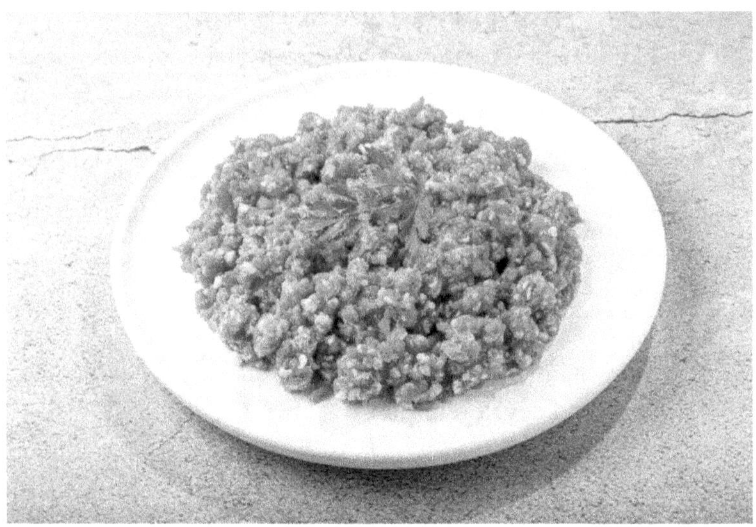

Satisfy your cravings with our savory Taco Pie. A perfect fusion of Mexican and American flavors, this pie features a hearty base of spiced meat and beans topped with a layer of melted cheese and crispy pastry. Indulge in this gluten-free option for a comforting and delicious meal.

Preparation Time: 45 min.

Serving Size: 4

Ingredients:

- 1 pound ground beef
- 1/2 cup of chopped onion
- 1/2 cup of chopped green bell pepper
- 1 package taco seasoning mix
- 1 can (8 ounces) of tomato sauce
- 1 can (8.5 ounces) of corn, drained
- 1 can (2.25 ounces) of sliced black olives, drained
- 1 cup of shredded cheddar cheese
- 1/2 cup of Bisquick baking mix
- 1/2 cup of milk
- 1 egg

XXXXXXXXXXXXXXXXXXXXXXX

Instructions:

a) Begin by preheating your oven to 400°F (200°C).

b) In a skillet, cook the ground beef, onion, and bell pepper over medium heat until the beef is fully browned and cooked.

c) Stir in the taco seasoning mix, tomato sauce, corn, and black olives. Continue to cook for an additional 5 minutes.

d) In a mixing bowl, combine the Bisquick baking mix, milk, and egg, stirring until the mixture is thoroughly combined.

e) Grease a pie dish and pour the cooked ground beef mixture into it. Sprinkle the shredded cheddar cheese evenly over the top.

f) Pour the Bisquick mixture over the cheese.

g) Bake the assembled pie in the preheated oven for approximately 30 minutes or until the crust turns a delightful golden brown.

h) Allow the Taco Pie to cool for a few minutes before serving.

Cooking Notes:

- Customize your Taco Pie by adding toppings like diced tomatoes, sliced jalapenos, or chopped cilantro for added flavor and freshness.
- For added spice and flavor, you can use hot taco seasoning mix or add some crushed red pepper flakes or hot sauce to the meat mixture.
- Ensure that the ground beef is well-drained after cooking to prevent the pie from becoming too greasy.
- If you prefer a thicker layer of the Bisquick crust, you can double the Bisquick baking mix, milk, and egg quantities in the recipe.
- This dish can be served with a side of sour cream, salsa, or guacamole for a complete Tex-Mex meal.
- Taco Pie is a hearty and satisfying dinner option that the whole family will enjoy.

My Words

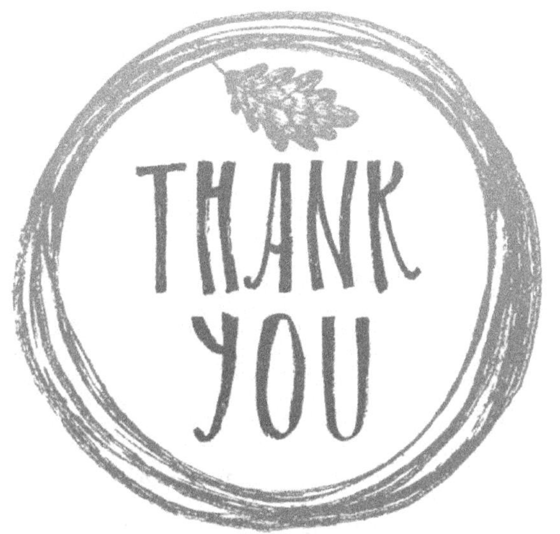

I cannot express enough how grateful I am for your decision to purchase my book. It is a humbling feeling to know that people are interested in learning from my experiences and the content that I have created. Being a writer has allowed me to share my knowledge and skills with others, and it is truly an honor to have you choose my book out of the multitude of books available on the market.

Your choice to invest in my book is incredibly special to me, and I am confident that the content you will find within its pages will prove to be valuable and insightful. It is my sincere hope that you will learn a great deal from the knowledge I have shared and that it will positively impact your life in some way.

After reading the book, I kindly request that you leave feedback, no matter how small. As a writer, I am always looking to improve and provide better content to my readers. Your feedback will be an invaluable source of information, and I will take it into consideration when creating future books. It is my goal to create content that my readers love and find helpful, and your input will play an important role in helping me achieve that.

Once again, I would like to express my gratitude for your support and for choosing my book. Your investment in my work means the world to me, and I am honored to have the opportunity to share my knowledge with you. Your feedback and support will be greatly appreciated and will help me to continue creating meaningful and valuable content for readers like you.

Kind regards,

Alex Aton